Malaria

By

Dr. Steve J. Hayes

Malaria

Copyright © by Dr. Steve J. Hayes 2023. All rights reserved. Before this document is duplicated or reproduced in any manner, the publisher's consent must be gained. Therefore, the contents within can neither be stored electronically, transferred, nor kept in a database.
Neither in part nor full can the document be copied, scanned, fixed, or retained without approval from the publisher or creator.

Table Of Contents

Malaria..1

Introduction 4

Chapter 1...5

What is malaria and how does it spread 5

Chapter 2...17

Leptospirosis 17

Chapter 3...32

Heat rash..32

Chapter 4...43

Prickly Heat (Miliaria Rubra)..43

Conclusion..52

Introduction

A parasite is the illness that causes malaria. Through mosquito bites carrying the parasite, people become infected. Malaria typically causes severe illness, including a high temperature and chills that cause trembling. Malaria is still widespread in tropical and subtropical nations, while being rare in temperate areas.

Chapter 1

What is malaria and how does it spread

Intestinal sickness is brought about by parasites that enter your body through the chomp of a contaminated mosquito. This occasionally deadly illness occurs in hot and damp spots, similar to Africa.

What is jungle fever?

Jungle fever is a serious illness that spreads when you're nibbled by a mosquito contaminated by little parasites. At the point when it nibbles, the mosquito infuses intestinal sickness parasites into your circulation system. Jungle fever is brought about by parasites, not by an infection or by a kind of bacterium.

In the event that it isn't dealt with, jungle fever can cause serious medical conditions, for example, seizures, cerebrum harm, inconvenience in breathing, organ disappointment, and passing.

Malaria

The illness is uncommon in the U.S., with around 2,000 cases each year. In the event that you're going to an area where jungle fever is normal, converse with your medical services supplier about ways you can forestall being contaminated. Individuals who are contaminated and travel to the U.S. can spread the infection in the event that a mosquito chomps them and, nibbles another person.

How normal is jungle fever?

Jungle fever is normal in tropical regions where it's hot and sticky. In 2020, there were 241 million detailed instances of jungle fever all through the world, with 627,000 passings because of jungle fever. Most of these cases happen in Africa and South Asia.

Where does intestinal sickness generally happen?

Jungle fever happens all around the world and happens most frequently in agricultural nations and regions with warm temperatures and high dampness, including:

- Africa.

- Focal and South America.
- Dominican Republic, Haiti, and different regions in the Caribbean.
- Eastern Europe.
- South and Southeast Asia.
- Islands in the Focal and South Pacific Sea (Oceania).

Who could get jungle fever?

Anybody can get jungle fever, yet individuals who live in Africa have a higher gamble of the disease than others. Small kids, more seasoned individuals and people who are pregnant have an expanded gamble of biting the dust from intestinal sickness. Individuals who live in destitution and don't approach medical care are bound to have complexities from the illness.

Over 90% of jungle fever passings happen in Africa, and practically individuals who bite the dust are all small kids. Over 80% of jungle fever passings in the locale in 2020 involved kids younger than 5 years of age.

Side Effects AND CAUSES

What causes intestinal sickness?

At the point when a mosquito nibbles somebody who has jungle fever, the mosquito becomes contaminated. At the point when that mosquito nibbles another person, it moves a parasite to the next individual's circulatory system. There, the parasites duplicate. There are five kinds of intestinal sickness parasites that can contaminate people.

In uncommon cases, individuals who are pregnant and who have jungle fever can move the sickness to their kids previously or during birth.

It's conceivable, however improbable, for intestinal sickness to be gone through blood bondings, organ gifts, and hypodermic needles.

What are the signs and side effects of intestinal sickness?

Signs and side effects of jungle fever are like influenza side effects. They include:

- Fever and perspiring.
- Cools that shake your entire body.
- Cerebral pain and muscle hurt.
- Weariness.
- Pain in the chest, difficulty breathing, and hacking.
- Loose bowels, sickness, and regurgitating.
- As jungle fever deteriorates, it can cause pallor and jaundice (yellowing of the skin and whites of the eyes).

The most serious type of jungle fever, which might advance to a state of insensibility, is known as cerebral intestinal sickness. This type addresses around 15% of passings in kids and almost 20% of grown-up passings.

When do side effects start on the off chance that you're tainted with jungle fever?

Jungle fever side effects as a rule seem 10 days to one month after the individual was contaminated. Contingent upon the sort of parasite, side effects can be gentle. Certain individuals don't feel wiped out for as long as a year after the mosquito nibble. Parasites can some of the time live in the body for quite some time without causing side effects.

A few sorts of jungle fever, contingent upon the kind of parasite, can happen once more. The parasites are latent in your liver and afterward are delivered into your circulatory system after years. The side effects start again when the parasites start flowing.

Determination AND TESTS

How is intestinal sickness analyzed?

Your medical care supplier will analyze you and get some information about your side effects and travel history. It's critical to share data about the nations you've visited as of late with the goal that your supplier can obviously grasp your gamble.

Your supplier will take an example of your blood and send it to a lab to check whether you have intestinal sickness parasites. The blood test will let your supplier know if you have jungle fever and will likewise distinguish the kind of parasite that is causing your side effects. Your supplier will utilize this data to decide the right treatment.

The executives And Treatment

How is intestinal sickness treated?

It's critical to begin regarding jungle fever at the earliest opportunity. Your supplier will endorse prescriptions to kill the jungle fever parasite. A few parasites are impervious to intestinal sickness drugs.

A few medications are given in blend with different medications. The sort of parasite will figure out what kind of prescription you take and how long you take it.

Antimalarial drugs include:

- Artemether and artesunate are artemisinin-based medicines. The best treatment for Plasmodium falciparum intestinal sickness, in the event that accessible, is artemisinin blend treatment.
- Atovaquone (Mepron®).
- Chloroquine. There are parasites that are impervious to this prescription.

Malaria

- Doxycycline (Oracea®, Monodox®, and Doxy-100®).
- Mefloquine.
- Quinine.
- Primaquine.

Drugs can fix your intestinal sickness.

What are the results of prescriptions to treat intestinal sickness?

Antimalarial medications can cause incidental effects. Make certain to enlighten your supplier concerning the different meds you're taking, since antimalarial medications can impede them. Contingent upon the drug, secondary effects might include:

- Gastrointestinal (GI) issues like queasiness and runs.
- Cerebral pains.
- Expanded aversion to daylight.
- A sleeping disorder and upsetting dreams.
- Mental issues and vision issues.
- Ringing in the ears (tinnitus).
- Seizures.

- Pallor.
- Avoidance

Might I at any point forestall jungle fever?

In the event that you anticipate residing briefly in or making a trip to an area where jungle fever is normal, converse with your supplier about taking meds to forestall jungle fever. You should consume the medications previously, during, and after your visit. Prescriptions can extraordinarily diminish the possibility of getting jungle fever. These medications can't be utilized for treatment assuming you in all actuality do foster jungle fever regardless of taking them.

You ought to likewise play it safe to keep away from mosquito nibbles. To bring down your possibility of getting jungle fever, you ought to:

- Apply mosquito repellent with DEET (diethyltoluamide) to uncovered skin.
- Wrap mosquito netting over beds.
- Put screens on windows and entryways.
-

Malaria

- Treat clothing, mosquito nets, tents, hiking beds, and different textures with a bug repellent called permethrin.
- Wear long jeans and long sleeves to cover your skin.

Is there an immunization against jungle fever?

There's an immunization for kids which was created and tried in Ghana, Kenya, and Malawi in an experimental run program. The RTS, S/AS01 immunization is compelling against Plasmodium falciparum jungle fever, which causes extreme illness in youngsters.

Different projects are attempting to foster intestinal sickness immunization.

Standpoint/Guess

What is the standpoint for individuals who have jungle fever?

On the off chance that intestinal sickness isn't dealt with as expected, it can cause significant medical conditions, including extremely durable organ harm and passing. It's vital to look for treatment immediately in the event that you assume you have jungle fever or have visited a region where it is normal. Treatment is significantly more compelling when it's begun early.

The right prescription and address portion can treat jungle fever and clear the disease from your body. Assuming you've had jungle fever previously, you can get it once more on the off chance that a tainted mosquito messes with you.

Living With

When would it be advisable for me to see my medical care supplier about intestinal sickness?

In the event that you've ventured out to or live in a nation where jungle fever is normal and you have side effects of intestinal sickness, see your supplier right away. The early finding makes treatment more viable. It's additionally vital to look for treatment immediately to prevent intestinal sickness from spreading to other people.

As often as possible Got clarification on pressing issues

Malaria

How is sickle cell attribute connected with jungle fever?

Throughout the long term, researchers have found that individuals with sickle cell characteristics have some assurance against the kind of jungle fever brought about by Plasmodium falciparum. It appears to be that the sickle state of the red platelets catches the parasites and assists with annihilating them. Concentrates on going on in a bid to figure out how to apply this data.

Sickle cell characteristic happens when you have one sickle cell quality and one ordinary quality. It's not equivalent to sickle cell infection. Sickle cell pallor is important for a gathering of blood problems known as sickle cell infection.

Note

Jungle fever is a difficult disease, however, you can do whatever it may take to forestall it. You can bring down your gamble of disease by shielding yourself from mosquito chomps and taking preventive meds. On the off chance that you're voyaging where jungle fever is normal,

Malaria

converse with your supplier a little while before you leave. This is particularly significant assuming you're pregnant.

Chapter 2

Leptospirosis

Leptospirosis is a sickness brought about by the microorganisms Leptospira. You can get leptospirosis in the wake of getting water or soil debased by creature pee (pee) in your nose, your mouth, your eyes, or a break in your skin. Leptospirosis can cause influenza-like side effects that can deteriorate into Weil's disorder, a hazardous sickness, in a few individuals.

What is leptospirosis?

Leptospirosis is a disease brought about by contamination with the microbes Leptospira. You can get tainted with Leptospira through scraped areas or cuts in your skin, or through your eyes, nose, or mouth.

Leptospirosis is a zoonotic sickness, and that implies it's communicated among creatures and people. You can get contaminated through:

- Direct contact with pee (pee) or conceptive liquids from contaminated creatures.
- Contact with sullied water or soil.
- Eating or drinking sullied food or water.

Who is most in danger of leptospirosis?

You can get leptospirosis regardless of where you reside, however, it's mostly considered normal in tropical regions and hotter environments with heaps of precipitation every year. You're at an expanded gamble for leptospirosis assuming you live in or travel to these areas, including:

- Oceania (Australia, New Zealand, and the Pacific Islands).
- The Caribbean.
- Portions of sub-Saharan Africa.
- Portions of Latin America.
- South and Southeast Asia.

Flare-ups of leptospirosis have happened in the U.S. in the wake of flooding in Hawaii, Florida, and Puerto Rico. Sporting freshwater exercises, particularly ones that put you in touch with tainted water for significant stretches of time, put you at expanded risk. This incorporates exercises that put your head submerged or make you swallow water (for example, wilderness boating, swimming, and sailing). Your gamble is significantly more noteworthy after weighty precipitation or flooding.

How normal is leptospirosis in people?

It's assessed that more than 1 million individuals overall get leptospirosis every year. Right around 60,000 of those bite the dust from it.

What are the periods of leptospirosis?

Leptospirosis comprises two stages: the leptospiremic (intense) stage and the insusceptible (deferred) stage. You might have gentle side effects or no side effects in the leptospiremic stage. Certain individuals foster extreme side effects in the resistant stage.

Malaria

Leptospiremic stage

During the leptospirosis stage (additionally called the septicemic stage) you might encounter an unexpected beginning of influenza-like side effects. This often starts two to fourteen days following a Leptospira infection.

It endures somewhere in the range of three and 10 days.

In this stage, microorganisms are in your circulation system and moving to your organs. Blood tests will give indications of disease.

Invulnerable stage

In the resistant stage, Leptospira microbes have moved from your blood to your organs. The microscopic organisms are most moved in your kidneys, which make pee (pee). Pee tests will give indications of the microbes and you'll have antibodies to Leptospira in your blood.

Few individuals will become exceptionally ill with Weil's condition in this stage. Weil's disorder causes interior death, kidney harm, and extreme yellowing of your skin and eyes (jaundice).

Side Effects And Causes

What are the side effects of leptospirosis in people?

Certain individuals have influenza-like side effects of leptospirosis and some have no side effects by any means. In extreme instances of leptospirosis, you have side effects of inward draining and organ harm.

In intense leptospirosis, side effects come on abruptly, including:

- High fever.
- Red eyes (conjunctival infusion).
- Cerebral pain.
- Chills.
- Muscle hurts.
- Stomach torment.
- Sickness and spewing.
- Loose bowels.
- (Jaundice) Yellow skin or eyes.
- Rash.

Extreme leptospirosis (Weil's disorder) side effects might begin three to 10 days after the fact, including:

Malaria

- Hacking up blood (hemoptysis).
- Chest torment.
- Inconvenience relaxing.
- Serious yellowing of your skin or eyes.
- Dark, falter crap (stool).
- Blood in your pee (hematuria).
- A decline in the sum you pee (pee).
- Level, red spots on your skin that seem to be a rash (petechiae).

What causes leptospirosis?

The microbes Leptospira cause leptospirosis. Microorganisms help your body through your mouth, nose, or eyes or through breaks in your skin. They make a trip through your blood to your organs, gathering in your kidneys (the organ that "cleans" your blood).

Your kidneys dispose of the superfluous or poisonous matter in your pee (pee). Microbes from your kidneys leave your body in your pee, which can spread leptospirosis to others or creatures.

Malaria

Leptospirosis spreads in what way?

Leptospira-containing animal urine is often how leptospirosis is transmitted to humans.

Practically any warm-blooded animal (like rodents, canines, ponies, pigs, or cows) can get leptospirosis. They might have not many or no side effects of the disease.

Creatures with leptospirosis can pollute water or soil (soil), which spreads the microbes to different creatures or people. Leptospirosis can be contracted from:

- Straightforwardly contacting pee or other body liquids from a creature with leptospirosis.
- Getting tainted water or soil in your eyes, nose, or mouth or in a break in your skin.

Many individuals can get leptospirosis immediately (an episode) after weighty rains and flooding. The floodwaters wash into waterways, lakes, and channels, carrying microscopic organisms with them.

Leptospirosis is seldom infectious starting with one individual and then onto the next.

Conclusion And Tests

How is leptospirosis analyzed?

Your medical care supplier determined leptospirosis to have an actual test, blood tests, and pee tests. Your supplier will get some information about your side effects, your movement history, and whether you might have been in touch with anything defiled. In the event that you're extremely wiped out, you might have a chest X-beam or CT check.

How tests will be analyzed leptospirosis?

Blood or pee tests. Your supplier will get a blood test from your arm with a little needle or you'll pee in a cup for a pee test. A lab will test the examples for indications of Leptospira.

Imaging. In the event that you are giving indications of serious leptospirosis, your supplier might utilize a chest X-beam, CT check, or other imaging. They'll utilize a machine to take photos of your body to search for harm to your organs.

Malaria

The board And Treatment

How is leptospirosis treated?

Your medical care supplier will treat leptospirosis with anti-infection agents. In the event that you have a gentle case, they might have you watch out for your side effects to check whether you seek better without treatment.

On the off chance that you have serious leptospirosis, you'll remain in the medical clinic. Your supplier will give you anti-infection agents straightforwardly through an IV (a needle associated with a cylinder that carries medication to your blood). Contingent upon which of your organs are impacted, you might require extra meds or systems.

What prescriptions and systems are utilized to treat leptospirosis?

Anti-toxins. Kinds of anti-toxins that treat leptospirosis incorporate doxycycline, amoxicillin, ampicillin, penicillin-G, and ceftriaxone. Your supplier will choose which to utilize in view of how debilitated you are and your clinical history.

Mechanical ventilation. In the event that your lungs are tainted with microbes, you might struggle to breathe and need the assistance of a machine to relax for you. Your supplier will give you medicine to keep you snoozing while you're associated with the machine.

Plasmapheresis. Likewise called plasma trade, plasmapheresis could help you assume you're in danger of organ harm from leptospirosis. During this methodology, your supplier eliminates your blood by utilizing a cylinder joined to a vein. A machine isolates your plasma from your blood and replaces it with a plasma substitute. Your blood is then gotten back to your body through another cylinder.

How would I deal with the side effects of leptospirosis?

For gentle side effects, your medical care supplier can prescribe therapies to assist you with feeling improved. Non-prescription drugs like ibuprofen (Advil®, Motrin®), naproxen (Aleve®), or acetaminophen

Malaria

(Tylenol®) can help a throbbing painfulness and diminish your fever.

Counteraction

How might I forestall leptospirosis?

An immunization for leptospirosis isn't accessible in the U.S. The most effective way to forestall leptospirosis is by not swimming or swimming in water that could have creatures pee in it. This incorporates floodwaters. Alternate ways you can decrease your gambling include:

- Taking precautionary medicine. Assuming you're voyaging and at a high gamble for leptospirosis, get some information about taking medicine to hold back from becoming ill (prophylaxis).
- Staying away from creatures that could have leptospirosis.
- Wearing defensive dress and shoes in the event that you work with or around creatures.
- Wearing defensive shoes and apparel assuming you must be in touch with water or soil that may be sullied with microorganisms.

- Staying away from water sports and swimming in lakes and streams after floods.
- Drinking just treated water. Try not to hydrate from lakes, waterways, and channels without bubbling it first.
- Wearing gloves assuming you need to contact dead creatures. Try not to contact them with your uncovered hands and clean up completely subsequently.
- Covering open cuts or wounds with a waterproof dressing.
-

Viewpoint/Anticipation

What could I at any point expect in the event that I have leptospirosis?

Most instances of leptospirosis are gentle and don't require treatment. Your medical care supplier will in any case watch out for your side effects.

Assuming your side effects deteriorate or you have new side effects, make sure to your supplier. Go to the trauma center on the off chance that you have any side effects of Weil's condition.

How long does leptospirosis endure?

Gentle instances of leptospirosis last a couple of days to half a month. Assuming that you have extreme leptospirosis, you can be in the medical clinic for around fourteen days. It can require a while to recuperate from extreme leptospirosis completely.

When could I at any point return to work/school?

Leptospirosis is seldom infectious from one individual to another, so you can return to work or school when you feel improved.

Could people at any point endure leptospirosis?

Indeed, you can endure leptospirosis. Most instances of leptospirosis have no side effects or have extremely gentle side effects that disappear all alone.

Just around 1% of individuals with leptospirosis get seriously sick with Weil's disorder. Weil's disorder is frequently destructive in the event that not treated or on the other hand assuming you postpone treatment. However, whenever treated immediately, it's probably you'll recuperate.

Living With

How would I deal with myself with leptospirosis?

Assuming you've been determined to have leptospirosis, watch out for your side effects. Contact your medical care supplier on the off chance that any of them deteriorate or on the other hand assuming you have new side effects.

When would it be a good idea for me to see my medical services supplier about leptospirosis?

Contact your medical care supplier assuming you've been in water or soil that might have been polluted with microbes and you have any side effects of leptospirosis.

Malaria

When would it be advisable for me to go to the trauma center?

Go to the closest emergency room on the off chance that you have side effects of extreme leptospirosis, including:

- Hacking up blood.
- Chest torment.
- Inconvenience relaxing.
- Yellow skin or eyes.
- Dark, falter crap (stool).
- Blood in your pee.
- A decline in the sum you pee.
- Rash-like red spots on your skin.
-

What inquiries would it be advisable for me to pose to my primary care physician?

How could I become ill?

When would it be advisable for me to circle back to you?

What side effects would it be a good idea for me to reach you about?

Malaria

When would it be advisable for me to go to the trauma center?

Note

Leptospirosis is an exceptional sickness that normally causes gentle side effects yet can cause difficult disease in a few individuals. It's critical to be aware assuming your work or side interests put you in danger, yet you don't have to hang up your kayak or work boots right now. Knowing your dangers, avoiding potential risks and perceiving side effects can assist with protecting you solid and any place life takes you.

Chapter 3

Heat rash

An intense rash regularly seems to be little clear, white, or red knocks on your skin. These knocks are now and again loaded up with liquid. They can show up anyplace that you sweat a ton, such as under the bosoms, the crotch, or the face.

What is heat rash?

Heat rash is a skin condition that frequently influences kids and grown-ups in blistering, moist weather patterns. You can foster intense rash when your pores become hindered and sweat can't get away.

A wide range of sorts of skin rashes exist. They can be unsettling, awkward, or tremendously excruciating. Heat rash is quite possibly the most well-known type.

Share on Pi

What in all actuality does warm imprudent resemble?

Various kinds of intensity rash can go in seriousness, and they all look somewhat changed.

Miliaria crystallina

This is the most well-known and mildest type of intensity rash. On the off chance that you have miliaria crystallina, you'll see little clear or white knocks loaded up with liquid on the outer layer of your skin. These knocks are air pockets of sweat that frequently exploded.

In spite of mainstream thinking, this kind of intense rash doesn't tingle and ought not to be difficult. Miliaria crystallina is more normal in youthful newborn children than in grown-ups.

Miliaria rubra

This sort, or "thorny intensity," is more normal in grown-ups than in youngsters and children. Miliaria rubra is known to cause more distress than miliaria crystallina on the grounds that it happens further in the external layer of the skin.

Miliaria rubra happens in hot or moist circumstances and may cause:

- bothersome or thorny sensations
- red knocks on the skin
- an absence of sweat in the impacted region
- aggravation and touchiness of the skin in light of the fact that the body can't deliver sweat through the skin's surface
- Knocks that show up because of miliaria rubra can once in a while advance and load up with discharge. At the point when this occurs, specialists allude to the condition as miliaria pustulosa.
-

Miliaria profunda

Miliaria profunda is the most un-normal type of intensity rash. It can repeat frequently and become constant, or long haul. This type of intense rash happens in the dermis, which is the more profound layer of skin. Miliaria profunda commonly happens in grown-ups after a time of actual work that produces sweat.

Assuming you have miliaria profunda, you'll see huge, extreme, tissue-shaded knocks.

Since heat rash keeps the sweat from leaving your skin, it might prompt queasiness and unsteadiness.

Treatment of intense rash

Heat rash typically settles without treatment in a couple of days. Assuming the uneasiness turns out to be excessively serious, you can attempt strategies at home that assist with relieving tingling and decreasing skin temperature.

A few medications/creams you can purchase to oversee heat rash include:

- Over-the-counter (OTC) hydrocortisone cream applied 1-2 times each day can assist with mitigating tingling.
- OTC allergy medicines can likewise produce a result against tingling.

Malaria

8 home solutions for heat rash

Besides OTC meds and creams, there are various natural or non-restorative cures that could calm the redness and tingling. These include:

- Apply a virus pack. Utilizing an ice pack or chilled material can assist you with cutting down redness, enlarging, and tingling. Assuming utilizing an ice pack, make certain to enclose it with a towel or old shirt — you would rather not experience cooler consumption.
- Wash up. A cold or tepid shower can likewise assist you with decreasing the temperature of your skin and calming tingling. It could assist with attempting an exfoliant to assist with opening the impacted pores.
- Maintain a cool interior temperature. Utilize a fan or cooling to chill off your room. In the event that you're on bed rest, it means quite a bit to move around to allow air to flow through your body.
- Stay with free, cotton clothing. This permits air to move around your body and keep it cool. Picking lightweight, breathable, normal textures instead of engineered materials could likewise assist you with

- keeping away from disturbance and remaining agreeable.
- Wash up. A 2015 studyTrusted Wellspring of colloidal oats extricate proposes that the conceivable mitigating and cell reinforcement impacts of oat may be behind its potential tingle calming impacts.
- Utilize effective pine tar. Involved by individuals overseeing skin conditions for millennia, applying pine tar to bothersome or kindled regions can diminish tingling and irritation.
- Apply Aloe vera gel to the area. Aloe vera is another deep-rooted effective solution for skin afflictions that might assist with relieving your bothersome skin.
- Blend sandalwood in with water and apply the glue to your intensity rash. A more seasoned 2011 investigation discovered that sandalwood, a spice normal to Ayurvedic conventional medication, could assist you with diminishing irritation across various skin conditions.
-

Side effects of intensity rash

Malaria

Heat rash frequently causes side effects in sweat-inclined regions, such as:

- the face
- the neck
- under the bosoms
- underneath your scrotum

The side effects can include:

- little raised spots called papules
- a tingling sensation
- slight expanding
- On lighter skin
- The spots might seem red.
- On more obscure skin
- The spots can be more downplayed and harder to recognize on hazier skin. In any case, a dermatologist or doctor will actually want to see them utilizing a dermoscopy, where they utilize a little, lit magnifying lens to focus on the skin.

For individuals with hazier skin, the spots could show up as white globules with more obscure radiances around them.

Malaria

What brings on a heat rash?

When pores are blocked from removing perspiration, heat rash develops.

This is bound to occur in hotter months or environments, or after serious activity.

Wearing specific kinds of apparel can trap sweat, prompting heat rash. Utilizing thick salves and creams can likewise prompt intense rash.

It's feasible to get heat rash in cooler temperatures assuming you wear garments or rest under covers that lead to overheating. Infants are bound to foster intense rash in light of the fact that their pores are immature.

Erosion on the outer layer of the skin frequently causes heat rash. Grown-ups typically foster intense rash on the pieces of their bodies that rub together, such as between the inward thighs or under the arms. Babies frequently foster intense rash on their necks, yet it can likewise foster skin folds like those of the armpits, elbows, and thighs.

Malaria

Risk factors

Having specific medical conditions or participating in a specific way of life decisions can expand your gamble for heat rash, including:

- being prone to excessive perspiring
- consistently captivating in extreme focus actual work
- ingesting medications that trigger perspiring like bethanechol, clonidine, and neostigmine
- Morvan condition, an uncommon hereditary issue that causes exorbitant perspiring
- type 1 pseudohypoaldosteronism, is a condition that causes a deficiency of sodium through the perspiration organs that has a connection to warm ill-advised
-

When would it be a good idea for you to call your PCP?

Heat rash is seldom serious. Frequently, it disappears without treatment in a couple of days. In any case, you ought to call your primary care physician assuming you start to encounter:

- a fever
- chills
- expanded torment
- discharge depleting from the knocks
- Call your kid's PCP in the event that your youngster has an intense rash that doesn't determine in a couple of days. Your primary care physician might suggest that you apply salves like calamine or lanolin to ease tingling and forestall further harm. Keep their skin cool and dry to assist with alleviating heat rash.
-

Counteraction

Follow these tips to forestall heat rash:

Abstain from wearing tight apparel that doesn't permit your skin to relax. Dampness-wicking textures might assist with forestalling sweat development on the skin.

Try not to utilize thick salves or creams that can obstruct your pores.

Do whatever it takes not to become overheated, particularly in hotter months. Search out cooling or convey a handheld fan.

Utilize a cleanser that won't dry your skin and doesn't have scents or colors.

The primary concern

Heat rash causes minor distress, spots, tingling, and expansion. It ordinarily sorts itself out surprisingly fast for a great many people. There are a few kinds that appear to be marginally unique from each other.

You can forestall it by remaining cool in hotter environments, wearing a free dress, and keeping away from thick creams.

Chat with your primary care physician assuming that you accept you might have something more serious or on the other hand on the off chance that you have an intense rash that regularly repeats.

Chapter 4

Prickly Heat (Miliaria Rubra)

What is thorny intensity?

The condition that we call thorny intensity happens to grown-ups and kids when sweat becomes caught under the skin.

It's likewise called heat rash, sweat rash, or miliaria rubra. Kids will quite often get it more than grown-ups in light of the fact that their perspiration organs are as yet creating.

Thorny intensity is awkward and irritated. Generally speaking, fostering the rash isn't a reason to the point of seeing a specialist. There are treatment choices and avoidance tips for individuals who oftentimes get thorny intensity.

Side effects of thorny intensity

The side effects of thorny intensity are genuinely direct. Red knocks and tingling happen in a space where sweat has been caught under layers of skin.

The neck, shoulders, and chest are the most well-known places for thorny intensity to show up. Folds of skin and where your dress rubs against your skin are additional regions where thorny intensity could happen.

The area of bothering could show a response immediately, or it could require a couple of days to foster on your skin.

At times thorny intensity will appear as a fix of tiny rankles. This is your skin's reaction to the sweat that seeps between its layers. At different times the region of your body where sweat is caught could seem enlarged or tingle industriously.

At times, an individual with thorny intensity may likewise foster pustules on their skin. This type of condition is known as miliaria pustulosa. This might demonstrate a bacterial disease.

Causes and triggers

Blistering climate, especially close by moistness, is the most well-known trigger for thorny intensity rash. Your body makes sweat to chill off your skin.

At the point when you sweat beyond what is regular, your organs can become overpowered. The perspiration channels might become hindered, catching the perspiration profoundly under your skin. The perspiration may likewise spill through layers of your skin near the epidermis, or top layer, and become caught there.

It's feasible to get thorny intensity whenever of year, however, it's mostly considered normal in the hotter months. Certain individuals who are utilized to cooler environments will quite often encounter heat rash when they travel to tropical spots where the temperatures are essentially higher.

Thorny intensity on a child

Youngsters, particularly babies, are particularly helpless against thorny intensity. Their perspiration organs aren't

Malaria

yet completely created, and their skin isn't utilized to quickly evolving temperatures.

Babies will generally encounter thorny intensity all over and in the folds of their skin around the neck and crotch.

Like most child rashes, thorny intensity is typically innocuous and will disappear all alone. Your child could act surly and be hard to relieve while they're encountering the bothersome vibe of intensity rash.

In the event that you notice a little fix of small red rankles underneath your kid's skin, assess their environmental factors.

Could it be said that they are wearing such a large number of layers? Is their clothing fitting for the temperature?

Is your child acting fretful, and does their pee show they could be dried out?

A cool shower will give help to your kid as a rule. Keep their skin dry when it's not shower time. Keep away from oil-based items, as they could obstruct the pores further.

On the off chance that your child shows a fever over 100.4°F (38°C) or different side effects, call their pediatrician.

Instructions to quiet the irritated or thorny inclination

Heat rash, including thorny intensity, will frequently disappear without therapy.

The initial step to relieving thorny intensity is to create some distance from the aggravation (or climate) that is making your skin break out in perspiration. When you're in a cooler climate, the vibe of tingling under your skin could require a long time to die down.

Different solutions for thorny intensity include:

- wearing light, baggy apparel
- staying away from skin items that contain oil or mineral oil
- keeping away from perfumed cleansers or body care items
- applying a virus pack, which you can make at home utilizing a plastic sack or towel

In certain cases, medical care proficient will suggest triamcinolone 0.1% cream (Triderm). This effective corticosteroid is just accessible by solution in the US. In the event that you have miliaria pustulosa, medical care proficient will recommend an effective anti-microbial, for example, clindamycin.

An assortment of over-the-counter (OTC) items are likewise accessible to assist with treating thorny intensity.

Over-the-counter (OTC) items

Calamine moisturizer is a characteristic solution for thorny intensity. It tends to be applied to the impacted region to cool the skin.

Different items to attempt include:

- OTC corticosteroids, for example, hydrocortisone cream in a low dose
- anhydrous lanolin, a waxy salve got from fleece
- effective or oral allergy medicines to decrease tingling

On the off chance that pricky intensity is related to fever, you might consider fever minimizers like ibuprofen

(Advil, Motrin) or acetaminophen (Tylenol). Talk with medical care proficient prior to giving one of these drugs to a kid.

Counteraction tips

The best method for staying away from thorny intensity is to avoid circumstances that cause unnecessary perspiring. Attempt these tips:

Wear baggy cotton clothing on the off chance that you realize you will be in a sweltering or damp environment.

Clean up or shower often in the event that you're visiting a warm or sticky environment.

In the event that you're in a sweltering or damp environment, put in a couple of hours every day in a cool space with fans or cooling.

Pick lightweight sheet material, for example, cotton or cloth sheets.

At the point when you practice outside, pick gear that will wick dampness away from your skin.

Malaria

Try to change out of sweat-soaked or wet apparel immediately subsequent to encountering serious intensity.

Change your child's diaper following they wet or soil it.

Remain very much hydrated by drinking a lot of liquids.

Viewpoint for thorny intensity

Heat rash typically disappears all alone. On the off chance that the rash is by all accounts deteriorating, or the region appears as though it's becoming contaminated, think about seeing a specialist.

Recall that microorganisms live in your skin. Inordinate tingling can make a painful injury that will become contaminated as you keep on contacting it.

Certain individuals have hyperhidrosis, a condition in which their bodies produce an excess of sweat. On the off chance that you suspect you're perspiring excessively, you might need to see a dermatologist.

Assuming you notice thorny intensity showing up on your skin, be aware of everything your body is attempting to

Malaria

say to you. Make a point to remain hydrated in warm environments and during active work.

Watch for different indications of intensity fatigue (like wooziness, migraine, or fast pulse) and move to a cooler region in a hurry.

Conclusion

You now have a better understanding of the United Against Malaria campaign's four pillars and some straightforward suggestions for staying malaria-free. Malaria, one of the oldest and deadliest illnesses that affect humans, can and ought to be eliminated by 2050. Under the status quo, malaria will not be eliminated. Actions that are specific and crucial are needed at To guarantee eradication, action must be taken at the national, regional, and international levels. You may advance your malaria preventionefforts with the aid of my book.

These materials are meant to complement your understanding on malaria and its prevention and control methods, not to replace it.

www.ingramcontent.com/pod-product-compliance
Lightning Source LLC
Chambersburg PA
CBHW070135230526
45472CB00004B/1546